YOUR KNOWLEDGE HAS VALUE

- We will publish your bachelor's and master's thesis, essays and papers

- Your own eBook and book - sold worldwide in all relevant shops

- Earn money with each sale

Upload your text at www.GRIN.com
and publish for free

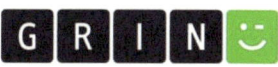

Anna Hudalla

Inequalities in Health

Which inequalities exist and why this is seen as a social problem

GRIN Verlag

Bibliografische Information der Deutschen Nationalbibliothek:

Die Deutsche Bibliothek verzeichnet diese Publikation in der Deutschen Nationalbibliografie; detaillierte bibliografische Daten sind im Internet über http://dnb.d-nb.de/ abrufbar.

Dieses Werk sowie alle darin enthaltenen einzelnen Beiträge und Abbildungen sind urheberrechtlich geschützt. Jede Verwertung, die nicht ausdrücklich vom Urheberrechtsschutz zugelassen ist, bedarf der vorherigen Zustimmung des Verlages. Das gilt insbesondere für Vervielfältigungen, Bearbeitungen, Übersetzungen, Mikroverfilmungen, Auswertungen durch Datenbanken und für die Einspeicherung und Verarbeitung in elektronische Systeme. Alle Rechte, auch die des auszugsweisen Nachdrucks, der fotomechanischen Wiedergabe (einschließlich Mikrokopie) sowie der Auswertung durch Datenbanken oder ähnliche Einrichtungen, vorbehalten.

Imprint:

Copyright © 2011 GRIN Verlag GmbH
Druck und Bindung: Books on Demand GmbH, Norderstedt Germany
ISBN: 978-3-656-54130-1

This book at GRIN:

http://www.grin.com/en/e-book/264756/inequalities-in-health

GRIN - Your knowledge has value

Der GRIN Verlag publiziert seit 1998 wissenschaftliche Arbeiten von Studenten, Hochschullehrern und anderen Akademikern als eBook und gedrucktes Buch. Die Verlagswebsite www.grin.com ist die ideale Plattform zur Veröffentlichung von Hausarbeiten, Abschlussarbeiten, wissenschaftlichen Aufsätzen, Dissertationen und Fachbüchern.

Visit us on the internet:

http://www.grin.com/

http://www.facebook.com/grincom

http://www.twitter.com/grin_com

University of Nottingham

School of Sociology & Social Policy

Inequalities in Health

Which inequalities exist and why this is seen as a social problem

Module Title: Health: Theory, Policy and Practice

Student ID: 2107790 (Erasmus student)

January 13th, 2011

Table of Contents

Abstract 1

How to assess Inequalities in Health 2

    Concept of Measuring Health 2

    Concept of Inequalities 2

    Concept of Social Class 3

Existing Inequalities 4

    Life Expectancy 4

    Infant Mortality 5

    Life Satisfaction 7

    Conclusion 9

Inequalities as a Social Problem 9

Table of Figures II

Bibliography III

Abstract

This essay is about inequities in health and to what extent they are seen as a social problem. In the first part the measurements for "inequalities" and "health" are clarified. Applying these measurements, the second part highlights currently existing inequalities in health in the UK today. The last part of the essay assesses the question why inequalities steam from social differences and what makes them problematic.

How to assess Inequalities in Health

In 1977, the working group of inequalities in health, known as the "Black Group", was given the task to review information about differences in health status between the social classes;...,' (Black, 1980: p.10). More than thirty years have passed since that first official assessment of the impact of social differences on the status of health. But still the question to reveal inequalities in health (the first part of the essay) is the same.

Concept of Measuring Health

Our understanding of what we perceive as health and ill-health is not a stable construct. It rather has varied throughout the past and according to experience, society and situational factors and each subgroups of the society will have a slightly different focus about how to understand health (Black, 1980: pp.12). In order to assess health and differences in health, our subjective constructs and understandings of health first need to be transferred into measurable, operational terms.

According to the Black report, the most common measurements of health are 'mortality rate, prevalence or incidence morbidity rates, sickness-absence rates and restricted-activity rates' (Black, 1980: pp.12). This essay will mainly focus on mortality rates which are in line with the Black report and a very familiar form of measurement. However each measurement has its own limitation and it should be mentioned that the major drawbacks of mortality rate is that it tends to underestimate the prevalence of chronic illness and other disease which influence human "well-being". Therefore it is critical to keep in mind other forms of assessment and combine those, for example a reflection of social, emotional and physical functions (Black, 1980: pp.12) such as the measurement of life satisfaction included into this analysis.

Concept of Inequalities

The term *inequality in health is* not simply a question of assessment as clarified above. Once we have identified how to measure health, we need to clarify what is understood by *inequalities*.

The Black report differentiates between *inequalities* and *differences*. Differences such as in race, sex or age are naturally occurring and therefore not seen as problematic. Inequalities however are 'brought about by social ... organizations and ... tend to be regarded as undesirable or of doubtful validity by groups of society` (Black, 1980: pp.16). Consequently it can be said that the Black report shapes the term both as resulting from *socio-economic* differences and as *morally not neutral*. This specific meaning should be carried in mind throughout the text. However not everybody appreciates the rather loaded and slightly ambiguous meaning of the term. Therefore the World Health Organization rather proposed the term `inequities` for inequalities which are unjustifiable and undesirable (Macintyre, 2002: p.210).

Concept of Social Class

Why is social class used as a measure and how is it constructed?

After assessing how to measure health we now need to define the second variable, a measure of inequalities. As the discussion on inequalities above suggests, it ought to be some kind of social-economic construct. In Britain, there has been a long tradition of measuring inequalities in health in terms of *occupational class* or status. This is dating back as long as the seventeenth century and was rather adopted by Black in 1980 then newly constructed (Macintyre, 2002: p.198). The widespread use of occupation can be accounted for by its comparable easy usage. As Black explains it,

> `inequalities are difficult to measure and trends in inequalities in the distribution of income and wealth, for example, cannot be related to indicators of health, except indirectly. Partly for reasons of convenience, therefore, occupational status or class (which is correlated closely with various other measures of inequality), is used as the principal indicator of social inequalities ….' (Black, 1980: p.14).

Occupational status is therefore strongly related to a wide range of other factors associated with inequalities such as housing, education, income-level and life-style. It will hence be used in the analysis. The Registrar General's Social Class (RGSC) of socio-economic classification is applied, although since 2001 the new National Statistics Socio-Economic Classification (NS-SEC), with up to eight occupational categories, has been introduced. (Office of National Statistics, 2010: p.1)

However in order to ensure that past statistics are correctly incorporate into the analysis of long-term trends, the following "old" classification system is used:

I.   Professional (e.g. accountant, doctor, lawyer) (5%)
II. Intermediate (e.g. manager, schoolteacher, nurse) (18%)
III. i) Skilled non-manual (e.g. clerical worker, secretary, shop assistant) (12%)
     ii) Skilled manual (e.g. bus driver, butcher, coal face worker, carpenter) (38%)
IV. Partly skilled (e.g. agricultural worker, bus conductor, postman) (18%)
V.   Unskilled (e.g. labourer, cleaner, dock worker) (9%)

(Source: Black, 1980 p.15)

Existing Inequalities

As we have defined the operational terms, we will now continue to reveal existing inequalities.

> "There is so much evidence demonstrating differences in mortality and morbidity between the social classes ... that it is difficult to select from evidence. These differences are well known." (Brotherston, 1975 quoted in Macintyre, 2002: p.203)

This quote was used as the opening sentence of a lecture on inequalities of health in 1975. Although the phrase seems outdated today, it clearly and sadly is not! There is a huge amount of research about social class differences in relation to health. However this article puts a lot of emphasis on using *recent* data and up-to-date information. On important construct needs to be introduced for a better understanding of the analysis: In November 2004 the Department of Health introduced the *Spearhead Group* which consists of the Local Authority areas that have the worst health and deprivation indicators compared to the rest of England. It contains 70 Local Authorities and the 62 Primary Care Trust areas they belong to. In total, the Spearhead group contains 28% of the population of England, more than a quarter (Health Inequality Unit, 2007: p.5).

Life Expectancy

The first indicator for inequalities is the age people are expected to reach. Nationwide life expectancy has increased in the last 20 years for both men and women and including the Spearhead areas. There has been an increase of 3,1 years for males and of 2,1 years for females in the population between 1995-'97 and 2005-'07. However the improvement in life expectancy is unequally distributed. For Spearhead areas there is less increase in life expectancy. Especially women in the Spearhead group have a lower level of improvement with only 1.9 years extra and with 2.9 years for males in the Spearhead areas (Department of Health, 2009: p.8). Although the difference of 0,2 years is only a slight deviation from the national trend, the gap in life expectancy between disadvantages areas and the rest remains wide with 2% for males and by 11% for females in 2004-'06 (Health Inequality Unit, 2007: p.7). This trend underpins the existing variation between social groups, displayed in the graph below, with people from the professional occupational class having the highest life expectancy with a descending trend according to the occupational classes (Department of Health, 2009: p.118, Health Inequality Unit, 2007: pp.3). However there are some exceptions to this trend. Between 1997-2001 life expectancy for man increased especially for group I., "manual worker", which closed the difference to the non-manual group. For woman, occupational group seems to be less influential as ´estimates of life expectancy increased by a similar amount for those classified to non-manual and manual occupations` (Department of Health, 2009: p.118).

Figure 1: Life expectancy at birth by social class (England and Wales, 1992-2005)

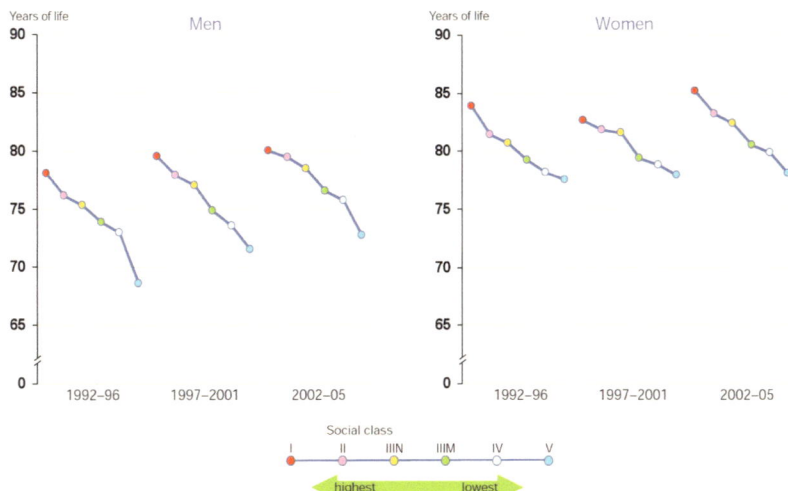

(Source: Department of Health, 2009 p. 117)

Infant Mortality

Infant mortality rate is seen as a ´good indicator of the health of a society´; the highly emotional component of infant death makes them especially critical and ´each avoidable death is one too many` (Health Inequality Unit, 2007: p.4). Infant mortality also heavily triggers the low life expectancy rates in the Spearhead group (Health Inequality Unit, 2007: p.4). Overall the Department of Health suggests in various publications that there has been a significant improvement in infant mortality over the past 10 years and that all social groups have been affected by the improving trend (Department of Health, 2009: pp.13). Please note, that unlike life expectancy rates, infant mortality is displayed in NS-SEC with three groups of the infants' parents. Those are I. "Managerial and professionals occupations", II. "Intermediate occupations" and III. "Routine and manual occupations". Further the groups "Other" (student, unemployed or people who never worked) and "Sole registrations" (children registered by the mother only) are added to the analysis (Office of National Statistics, 2010, Department of Health: p.1, 2009: p.118).

As the Department of Health relieved in 2008 (in the Status Report on the Program for Action) infant mortality was at an historic low level. Between 2005-'07, 4.7 infants per 1,000 live births died for all those in England with a valid socio-economic group compared to 5.6 per 1,000 in 1995–'97. (Department of Health, 2008: p.8). However, as can be drawn from the table below, there are still large differences between the occupational groups. For the routine and manual group there seems to be a recent narrowing in the gap between the rest of the population. In the last two years of assessment, 2004 to 2006, infant mortality rate was 17% higher in the routine and manual group than for the rest of the population, compared to of 18% in 2003-'05 and 19% in 2002-'04. However if evaluated against a difference of only 13% in 1997-'99 (Health Inequality Unit, 2007: p.5), it is questionable if there is much of an improvement. Further the disadvantage of the Routine and Manual group can be expressed in total numbers. In 2004 to 2006 there were 8,674 infant deaths in total. The Routine and Manual group accounted for 43% of them, creating a rate of 5.6 deaths per 1,000 live births. This is higher than the rate of 4.8 deaths per 1,000 for the other occupational groups combined (Health Inequality Unit, 2007: p.4). In the diagram below the group "Other "displays the highest mortality rate. However, in total this group accounted for only 9.4 per cent of the deaths in 2004-'06 (Department of Health, 2009: p.119).

Figure 2: Infant mortality rate by socio-economic group (England and Wales, 1996-2006)

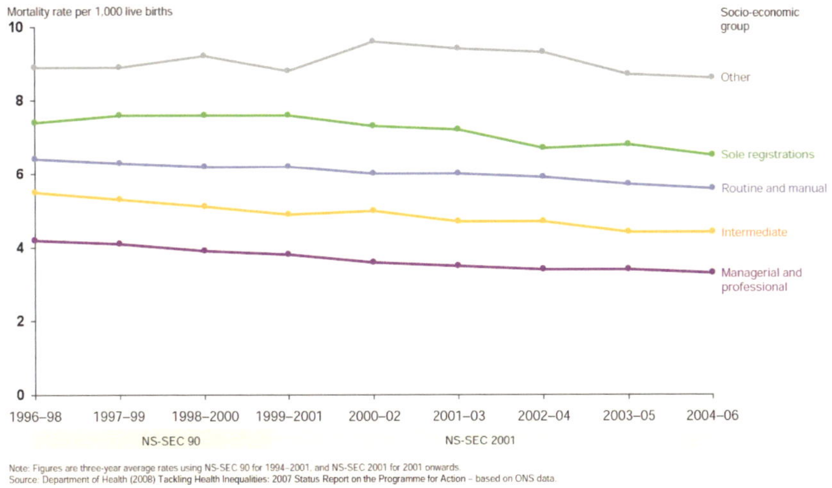

(Source: Department of Health, 2009 p.119)

Life Satisfaction

As mentioned in the introduction a measure of other factors besides mortality rates is critical in order to achieve an overview on existing inequalities. Therefore a measure of self-reported life satisfaction is included which was carried out by the Department of Environment, Food and Rural Affairs in 2007. Participants rated their life satisfaction on a scale from 1, least satisfied, to 10, most satisfied. They found that `approximately three-quarter (73 per cent) of the people in England rated their satisfaction with life as 7 or more out of 10` as depict in the graph below (Department of Health, 2009: p.111). In general there were high differences between both occupational group and age.

People in unskilled jobs, on state pension or unemployed were less satisfied with all aspects of their life compared to the other groups. On the other hand those people were more likely than average to have experienced negative feelings as depression, unsafe and lonely in the two weeks prior to the survey. On the other hand people in skilled jobs were had experienced feelings of happiness, energy and engagement with their activities in the same time period. When looking at the satisfaction rating, differences between occupational classes can be seen. There is a "social grading" applied in the given graph, which is determined by occupation. For that, Group AB with jobs like doctors, accountants, nurses or police officers, have an average satisfaction rating of 7.6. If compared to group E, which are unemployed, state pensioners or casual labours (rating 6.7) there is a decreasing trend. Ratings of a scale of 7 or 8, which are seen as having a satisfied life, were significantly less in this group, but ratings of 5, being neither satisfied nor unsatisfied, were more common than in group AB (Department of Health, 2009: p.111). It remains difficult to analyse the numbers in the same way as with e.g. infant mortality. Still a trend in differences in life satisfaction is seen. Besides the life satisfaction, social differences can also be seen in how people experience their own health. People in higher social classes generally consider their current health to be better. Further 76 % of those in a higher social class also expected to be in good health over a period as long as 10 years, compared to only 53% in the lowest social class (National Health Service, 2004: p.10). This and the satisfaction ratings clarify that inequalities do not only have impact on physical health but, maybe to a similar degree, also on psychological health. The reverse relationship holds true as well. There is a causal relationship between psychological life stress factors and poor health, as specifically chronic stress lowers the body's ability of regeneration and defence (Wilkinson, 1996: pp.175).

Figure 3: Self-reported life satisfaction by social grade (England, 2007)

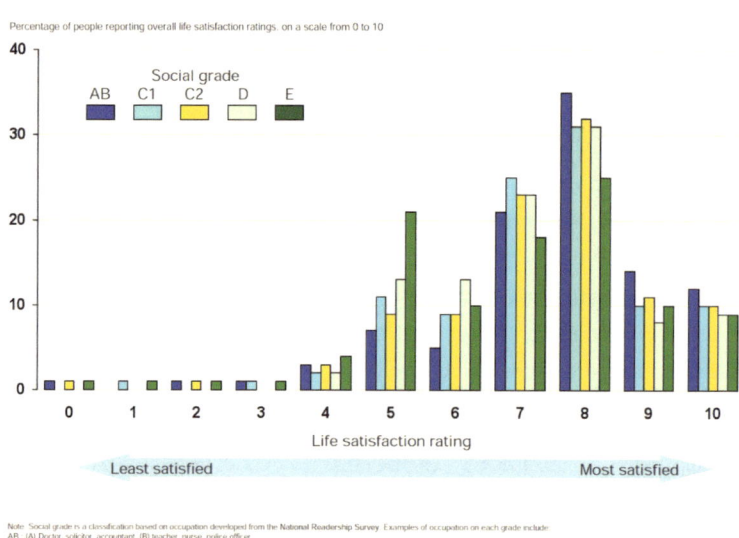

(Source: Department of Health, 2009 p.111)

Conclusion

The health of the population has significantly improved over the last 10 years, and this applies much the same for the disadvantaged groups and areas, as measured by life expectancy and infant mortality (Department of Health, 2009: pp.117). Although the infant mortality rates have declined, there is still need for improvement. On the one hand `each avoidable death is one too many and the number of pre-term babies is still too high`. And on the other hand, beside infant mortality, there are still a high number of children with long-term health conditions which embodies huge emotional and financial burdens for the families as well as for the government and society (Health Inequality Unit, 2007: p.4). An important part of social inequality is the psychological impact of it, which has a life-long effect. This impact should not be underestimated.

Inequalities as a Social Problem

Having assessed examples of the existing inequalities in the UK today, we now turn to the question why these differences are seen as a social problem. At first it is explained why inequalities are seen as a *social* issue, rather than an individual.

Much information can be found by looking at the results of the different reports on inequality in health. All documentation show similar causes. Starting with the Black Report (1980), a causal link was seen between social and economic factors and ill health. Namely, those factors were income, unemployment, poor environment, poor housing and education (Black, 1980: pp.158). The same results were confirmed by the Health Divide (1987) and the Acheson Report (1998). Out of those factors, the main causes of inequalities in health were poverty and education. The difference between the rich and the poor in a country and the differences between higher or lower education are socially influenced, constructed and maintained. Due to that, their impact on health is regarded as a social problem. A further influence stems from the role of the NHS. It has been shown that the impact of the NHS to health differences is relatively low, leaving the reasons for inequalities to other, social, problems (Department of Health, 2009: p.114).

In general, nowadays a grater deal of attention is devoted to the social and psychological consequences of low income. As the living standards have improved throughout the society, the effects of material privation are drastically reduced. Poverty is no longer seen as absolute (material privation) but as relative, compared to the rest of the society. Further the impact of poverty is redefined as ´social exclusion´ (Wilkinson, 2005: p.11). This clearly shows the social implication of low occupational groups. As a conclusion, it can be said that inequalities in health are seen as being social in their origin.

What still needs to be assessed is the question why those differences are (automatically) regarded as *problematic*. For most of us, inequalities are intuitively seen as unfair, wrong and problematic. This is especially true when they are itemized by social class as in the previous analysis. But why exactly are differences in health seen as a problem, while other differences in society such as income level or education level are more readily accepted and less viewed as problematic?

Obviously, a major reason is the outcome (or the consequences) of inequalities in health. Differences in the life expectancy means ´loosing loved ones earlier´ for a lower social group (Health Inequality Unit, 2007: p.5) as well as having a shorter life oneself. The same is true for infant mortality. The list of measurements of poorer health in lower social classes not assessed in this essay is long. Such are inequalities in lung cancer rates, cardiovascular diseases, accidents and suicides, respiratory diseases or obesity (Department of Health, 2009: pp.121). All of those health factors led to worse outcomes the lower the social class. As a result, those in a lower class have to deal with an enormous numbers of negative consequences, or put simple, bad health of themselves and relatives. The outcome in terms of health therefore builds the first reason to seen inequalities as problematic. However, the consequences relieve only half of the injustice. In lower social classes there is a higher prevalence of social and psychological factors such as stress, anxieties or depression. So the lives in the lower classes are on the one hand shorter due to worse medical conditions. And on the other hand they are less joyful, more filled with stress factors. Wilkinson calls this a bubble inequality as ´life is short where its quality is poor´ (Wilkinson, 2005: p.18).

In addition to the outcomes of poor health the major reason why inequalities are seen as a problem stems from the development of social classes. For children, social class is determined by the parents and changing the social class throughout one's own lifetime is difficult to achieve and in many cases it is not possible. Inequalities start before birth (smoking during pregnancy, children vaccine), at an age where the individual does not have any influence at his or her own lifestyle. Although randomly being born into one or the other social class does not display any injustice per se. But the fact that from the early beginning life is determined by a social construct, a social injustice where the individual does not have any influence on, is unfair. And therefore it is also problematic.

Generally inequalities in health due to social class are both socially *unfair* and *problematic*. Health inequalities effect major parts of the population (remember, 28% of the population is in the Spearhead Group). The well-being of the entire population can therefore only be improved through *major social changes.* That way, it can be achieved what the World Health Organization, calls "Health": A "state of complete physical, mental, and social well-being and not merely the absence of disease or infirmity" (Black,1980: p.10)

Table of Figures

Figure 1: Life expectancy at birth by social class (England and Wales, 1992-2005) 5
Figure 2: Infant mortality rate by socio-economic group (England and Wales, 1996-2006) ... 7
Figure 3: Self-reported life satisfaction by social grade (England, 2007) 8

Bibliography

Black, D., Morris, J., Smith, C. and Townsend, P. (1980) *Inequalities in Health: Report of a Working Party*, London: Department of Health and Social Security.

Department of Health (2008) *Tackling Health Inequalities: 2007 Status Report on the Program for Action*, Report, London: Department of Health

Department of Health (2009) *Tackling Health Inequalities: 10 Years On – A review of developments in tackling health inequalities in England over the last 10 years*, Report, London: Department of Health

Health Inequality Unit, Department of Health (2007) *Tackling Health Inequalities: 2004-06 data and policy update for the 2010 National Target*, Report, London: Department of Health

Macintyre, S. (2002) ` Before and After the Black Report: Four Fallacies`, in Berridge, V. and Blume, S. (eds) *Poor Health: Social Inequalities before and after the Black Report*, London: Frank Cass, pp 198-219

National Health Service (2004) *Choosing health: Making health choices easier*, Cm 6374, London: Stationery Office

Office of National Statistics (2010) `NS-SEC classes and collapses`. Available at http://www.ons.gov.uk/about-statistics/classifications/current/ns-sec/cats-and-classes/ns-sec-classes-and-collapses/index.html [Accessed 8th December 2010]

Wilkinson, R. G. (1996) *Unhealthy Societies: The Afflictions of Inequality*, London: Routledge

Wilkinson, R. G. (2005) *The Impact of Inequalities: How to make sick societies healthier*, London, Routledge